My Journey Through Rhinoplasty –
What I didn't know

By A.E. Sullivan

February 2013

Table of Contents

Introduction

I never really thought much about my nose. It was never my favorite facial feature, but neither was it tragic. It simply existed as part of given face.

When I was 15, my parents took me to an Ear, Nose, and Throat (ENT) specialist. I was having a whole stream of symptoms and my General Practitioner (GP) couldn't pinpoint a cause for my symptoms. I think initially the suggestion of seeing an ENT was just to start ruling out all possible systems in the body as the culprit. The ENT was local, and we only saw him once; I have to confess I don't remember his name or even what he looked like other than he had dark hair. The meeting was relatively short and uneventful – our two takeaways were 1) whatever my current problem was, the ENT did not think it was attributed to any of my E, N or T functions, and 2) my nasal cavity was blocked more than 50% on the left, and at least 10% on the right. (I think the blockage was the fault of my older sister – she ran me into the coffee table when I was 7 and the cartilage in my nose cracked noticeably – though it wasn't broke, and my nose hasn't been the same since. My sister claims it's not her fault.)

I gave my nose little thought after that. Sure, breathing through my nose was always a challenge, but it didn't seem to impact my life all that much. My teens gave way to my twenties and thirties my nasal cavities continued to narrow and I compensated more and more by simply breathing through my mouth.

However, past couple of years I haven't felt quite right – short of breadth, lightheaded at times, and sleeping became a challenge. I also started running on a lot of adrenaline even in normal circumstances. We tried to addresses pieces of the greater picture through sleep aides, natural hormonal rebalancing, exercise, and homeopathic supplements. While some progress was made, I just didn't feel right.

In working with my naturopath, Dr. Midori Nishida – a wonderful and insightful naturopath with The Essence in Santa Monica, CA, we found that I had adrenal fatigue and that my body's circadian rhythm looked more like an artistic interpretation of a "V" than a stepped-decline, as it should. Putting the different pieces together, and in talking it through with my husband, we came to the conclusion that my body was in a perpetual "fight or flight" adrenal high giving me jitters and causing my insomnia, which was also contributing to my lightheadedness. Further, the perpetual "fight or flight" was being caused by my body's inability to get enough oxygen – basically because my nasal cavities were constricted, the airflow was blocked and I couldn't breathe naturally through my nose. This was especially problematic at night. Basically, my body was suffocating and was then panicking, only it was a perpetual situation.

While I am not a typical fan of Western medicine, medication or surgery, the path to wellness seemed pretty clear to me – I needed to have my nose surgically reconstructed or unblocked, however that was to happen in order to be able to breathe again and restore my body's natural functioning.

Not one to hesitate, I immediately researched the nasal conditions, finding the description and top doctor that specialized in what it sounded like what I thought was wrong with my nose – internal nasal blockage. I made an appointment in mid-June 2012 to see Dr. Timothy Smith, Director of the Oregon Sinus Center at Oregon Health and Science University in Portland, Oregon. So, mid-June up to OHSU my husband and I went for what turned out to be a four-hour series of tests and appointments, all conducted very thoroughly but efficiently. While there, I had a cat-scan of my nose, met with Dr. Smiths assistant for a primary diagnosis, met with Dr. Smith, and Dr. Smith brought in Dr. Michael Kim, from OHSU's Division of Plastic and Reconstructive Surgery, who also agreed to meet with us at the last minute. (Apparently my nasal cavity was blocking airflow in three different spots and required two different surgeries that could be done together.) Oh, and we also agreed to the surgery and signed pre-op papers that day! (Our options were pretty clear and hesitating or additional pondering wasn't going to change the action plan.) These people did not mess around!

On August 9th I had nasal surgery. One year post surgery, I can mostly breathe easily and clearly through my nose and my body has rebalanced its natural circadian rhythm. (At six months, my breathing was completely clear, I believe some of the blockage has grown back since then as I can feel the interference when I try to breathe deeply though my nose.) I am also sleeping naturally, without prescription sleep aides and I am learning to "breathe" again. However, my nose is still sensitive to touch, wearing sunglasses for extended periods can cause my nose to hurt and the skin on my nose is still "hard" or stiff, all side-effects the doctors said would persist for up to a year.

While the surgery was certainly a success, and I believe the attending physicians and their staff were superb, the journey through this process was not always easy and I felt unprepared for both surgery and the recovery. This is my journey through rhinoplasty – how I prepared, what questions I had, how I recovered and things I would do differently to prepare and recover if only I knew – what I wish someone would have told me. I hope this helps you on your journey.

My own personal disclaimer... I am not a physician and have no medical training, nor do I have scientific evidence or case studies that demonstrate the relationship between the steps I took to prepare for my surgery, and their impact on surgical recovery. What I did was based on my own personal beliefs and my experiences. I do believe though that the steps I took helped me prepare and recover from surgery though and helped my body to heal. Do your own research, do what feels right for you. This is what was right for me.

The following sections or chapters were initially intended to be blog posts, however, once I started writing my husband and I realized we had way more words that the average blog and opted instead to format this into a short book. The entries take the reader through the preparation for surgery, 30 days prior to my surgery until six months post surgery. These were all written at the time they state, so all text is written in the present tense.

Pre-Op Prep: Four Days and Counting

Today is Sunday, August 5th. In four days, I have rhinoplasty surgery to correct a deviated septum and internal structural blockage to my nasal cavity in hopes of being able to breath semi-normally for the first time in 30-odd years.

I am female, 40, married with two boys - 7 and 9. I am an investigator by nature and a researcher by training. At 38, this will be my fifth surgery – two arthroscopic knee surgeries in high school, Lasik eye surgery in my late 20s, and a necessary hysterectomy three years ago.

Surgery is not something my husband and I consider lightly; for me, this feels like a **big** event – a big scary, nerve-wracking event. I am optimistic about the outcome, however, I am too bogged down in the stress and anxiety of being "put to sleep" under general anesthesiology and "getting through" this with optimal outcomes to be anything closely related to excited.

My pet peeve going into this surgery, as with my previous ones, is that I feel unprepared for the surgery itself, let alone feeling like an empowered participant in my own health and healing, via the surgery, pre-op prep and post-op recovery. Have I mentioned that I am, in general, not a fan of traditional medicine, doctors or hospitals?

Through our own life journey, my husband and I have become more a naturalists and fans of homeopathic treatment. Despite being raised in households with traditional medicine focuses, we tend to gravitate towards more natural solutions and believe that, for the most part, our body is a natural tool and made to heal as such – our children were both born out of the hospital, we have annual check-ups for the whole family with a naturopath, we regularly seek homeopathic and food-based solutions to ailments, buy organic, have largely gluten and dairy-free diets and tend to seek out nature-based solutions. Having said that, there are times and uses for traditional medicine with its cutting edge technologies and amazing fixes for the body – we haven't found a natural alternative to nasal reconstruction surgery, so off to general anesthesiology I go.

However, as natural investigator and trained researcher, not to mention a conservative mom, I want to be as prepared for surgery as possible – a partner in my healing as much as I can be while unconscious on the operating table. Additionally, I emotionally need to feel some level of control and empowerment while being relatively helpless "under the knife". So began our journey towards pre and post-op prep.

First, we chose our doctor carefully. I researched, largely via the Internet, what I thought my problem was and who was the best doctor, relatively locally, to address this problem. (We are happy with the education and experience of the doctor we have chosen, or we would have widened our search out of state.) Also, on a personal note, when I had Lasik eye surgery, my family optometrist suggested the Lasik eye surgeon just 20 minutes or so away. My husband and I drove by the surgeon's office – it had a neon sign in the window. Sorry, but I'm not having surgery conducted by anyone who has a neon sign outside their office building – no how, no way under any circumstances. So, no neon signs for us. (Thank you Dr. Caster, the doctor we did see for Lasik. It's nearly 20 years later and my vision is still 20/20!)

We chose Dr. Timothy Smith, Director, Oregon Sinus Center. Ok, no personal references or referrals, but as Director of Oregon Health and Science University, Oregon Sinus Center, Dr. Smith's experience and interest profile matched my problem – and who better to talk to then the head of noses! So, first off, no middle manning, we sought after and chose the most senior experienced and specialized physician we could find. As it turns out, to properly fix my nasal blockage specifically, it is going to require the top two doctors in their field – one specializing in the interior of the nose – Dr. Smith and one specializing on the exterior – Dr. Michael Kim, Facial and Plastic Reconstructive Surgery.

Two short appointments and a CT scan, four short hours later we are on the docket for upcoming surgery – wow, these people do not mess around. A bit of a whirlwind, though a short one, but why delay right? We identified the problem and found the top doctor(s) to fix the problem, so time to get on with the fixing. (Ok, I didn't take it all quite that easily. It was really overwhelming, but I couldn't find fault in either the doctors' logic or conclusions, nor my own; we identified the problem, identified the limited solutions and picked the most effective next step. So after a couple of minutes of discussion with my husband who accompanied me to the appointments, we signed the surgical consent forms.)

Ok, so, step one is accomplished – find the best at what you need done to maximize your odds of optimal outcomes. Check.

So, doctors picked, insurance cleared, surgery scheduled, childcare arranged. Now what? We have a pre-operation appointment with both the doctors and the hospital team the day before my surgery – hours before really, but in the meantime, what do we do? How do I become a partner in Western/traditional medicine and seek my own optimal outcomes while going through surgery and recovery? It was a question unaddressed by the accomplished doctors or their staff. (Though I have to confess, I did not ask about preparing for surgery in our initial (and only) meeting before scheduling surgery as I was so overwhelmed by initial appointments and agreeing to surgery after just four hours.)

We were left feeling unprepared and unempowered, even though really all the doctors require of us is that I show up (and pay). For many, this is probably enough – be on time and adhere to their pre-op instructions - no excessive Vitamin E before surgery, no St. John's Wort and some other herbal remedies two weeks prior and no food after eight o'clock the night before. For us, those rather spare instructions left us feeling helpless. There must be more we can do to optimize the experience.

So as a researcher, my journey started with research. What was recommended for post-op recovery for rhinoplasty? How did you prepare for this surgery? What should my recovery expectations be? Many hours of Internet research later, the recommendations came down to the following simple instructions:

- Begin Bromelain, a natural pineapple enzyme, one week before surgery and continue for 2-4 weeks after,
- have Arnica, a natural substance for speeding the healing of bruises and pains, at the ready for after surgery, and
- have ice packs at the ready. This took some additional research, with the top rated I could find being Swiss Therapy Eye Mask (for post-surgery recovery).

Also mentioned, though not regularly in blogs and articles – make sure to drink fluids regularly after surgery, keep sodium levels low, and green tea is not proven effective, though some people say it may help.

Okay, easy enough. But this still didn't feel sufficient. What else could I do to aid my body's recovery? We go to great lengths to make our lives the best we can, and it still seemed like there should be more. How would I feel and what would I feel like doing? What else can I do to help make sure I heal the best I can and make my recovery as easy possible. I realize the medical staff cannot tell patients exactly how they will feel as everyone is different and every patient has a different life style and heals differently, but it would have been nice to know how some people did. I was able to find on Google images pictures of people post-rhinoplasty, but I don't know what the time frames were or how they felt. So, not a lot of help there. In the midst of the information age, I felt I was really starting from scratch. How can I get my body in the best possible shape for surgery?

So began my journey into pre-op prep...

First – get in shape! I had extra encouragement from a college friend (thank you Rachel – citrusflats.com) who had recently completed The Beach Bodies Insanity exercise program and Shakeology diet (and then became a Beach Bodies coach). Rachel posted a picture of her post-two kid body - she looks fantastic! And I have to confess that after the pregnancy and birth of my two boys, I never quite got my body back. It wasn't bad, just 8 pounds heavier than before I was pregnant, but I have still been carrying around some the extra pregnancy weight and have lost some of my earlier muscle and endurance. So the first order of business was to get in shape.

With that decision made just four weeks before surgery, I don't anticipate I'll achieve Rachel-like abs, I think I have farther to go than she did in the muscle department, but still working at it. With my husband's support, we started Shakeology together, as well as Gaiam Cardio Wake Up workouts every other day, and he coached me in adding interval training on my bike trainer every other day as well. This exercise plan is not a crazy start, but I felt I needed to build up my endurance before I took on more. Also, as a mom of two younger boys on summer break, this felt achievable. After two weeks of exercising every other day, I changed it to exercising three days and then taking an off day - 3 on, 1 off for the last two weeks before my surgery.

Now, with less than one week until surgery, my weight is only down a pound or two but I have lost an inch or so around my torso and have gained noticeable muscle tone. This is longer term lifestyle change that will continue; I haven't gotten as far pre-surgery as I would like to, but I believe this has helped my body be in better shape and will help with my recovery. In-shape – half a check?

When I prepped for my hysterectomy, a trusted Emergency Room doctor (and my uncle) recommended taking HGH – Human Growth Hormone – starting one week before my surgery and for three weeks after. He utilized this strategy when he had surgery on his arm, and had other patience do this as well, and had an impressive outcome. While not inexpensive (~$560), we felt this was a factor in the success for my hysterectomy and therefore also wanted to prep my body for the rhinoplasty with HGH – so we did. A week before my surgery, I began at-home shots of HGH and will continue daily until three weeks after surgery. HGH – check, in progress.

One of the Shakeology claims is that it helps detox your system. I don't know how you look inside your body and double check this, but I think having your body as free of toxins as possible normally, and especially before something like surgery, is important. So, in addition to the Shakeology, but also for relaxation and healing, I started making sure I got in the sauna at least twice a week, starting one week before surgery. Seven years ago for my birthday, my husband bought me a sauna – a two person (really one person) ultra-violet sauna. It was such a wonderful surprise and has been a great asset to our health. My uncle, the ER doc, (yeah Uncle Don) has told me many times that whenever he starts to feel a cold or something coming on, he jumps in the sauna. My husband and I, and often my sister or friends, has followed suit and jumped in our sauna. I love our sauna! Not only does it help "sweat out the bad stuff", it also does wonders on sore and tense muscles. A luxury I never thought of owning, but my husband bought in on e-bay, drove an hour to get it and assembled it himself as a surprise. I still don't know what he paid for it, but we both consider it well worth the investment and have counseled others to consider this as well. So, with sweat rolling off the body, sauna – check, in progress.

Water Intake. One of the blogs mentioned that it was important to have regular fluid intake after surgery. (My interpretation of this was that the author probably didn't mean wine, but....?) However, in thinking about this, it didn't make sense to me to just maintain high water intake levels post surgery. If water is an essential element in our body (and I'm pretty sure there is no debate on this one), wouldn't it be of greater benefit to ensure that water intake is high before surgery to help keep the body fluid, with toxins flushed out and be overall better for you? With obviously no scientific backing on this, my gut instinct told me to start checking my water intake levels. However, I don't really like water, I find the stuff makes me feel full and bloated – I've been told to only drink negatively charged ionic water but don't make a habit of buying bottled water – so this one took some creativity. For a while I was drinking lots (read 8 -12 cups) decaffeinated pear ginger tea – made really weak and with a little bit of raw sugar. However, after a while, while the tea tastes good my back started to ache and it didn't feel like my body was terribly happy with me, so one week before surgery I changed over to carbonated water (we have a home Soda Club water carbonator) and one tablespoon of Torani Vanilla Bean Syrup in a 32 ounce glass; I drink four to six of these a day. So, adequate water intake – Check, working on it and will continue.

I started seeing a chiropractor after I was rear-ended in a car accident ten years ago. Since then, I have seen three different chiropractors, all with different approaches, all helpful and all with something different to add. I see a chiropractor every three months or so, more often when there is something "going on". I saw a chiropractor regularly in preparation for the birth of my second son, and in preparation for my hysterectomy. This is one of those things that I can't always look inside my body and see the difference, though I certainly notice when things are off and I can't move my neck and the chiropractor makes my able to move, but I believe make sense. So, even if I wasn't tight or misaligned prior to my surgery (although I was), I would see the chiropractor in prep for any surgery.

Logically to me, if the hose is kinked (your spine), the blood, oxygen and nerve message flow is interrupted. To me, those interruptions can't be good or allow for optimal performance, so in preparation for my rhinoplasty, I started seeing a chiropractor one week before my surgery to make sure my spine was in alignment and would stay there until my surgery. I saw the chiropractor twice before my surgery and considered a third appointment, however the chiropractor did not think it was necessary. Chiropractic Care – Check, got my clean bill of health as of two days ago from the chiropractor. (Thank you Dr. Seth Fortier for the alignment and Michele for the recommendation. Also thank you Dr. Gina Caserma who educated me and advocated continually for regular chiropractic care.)

Along the same lines as detox and general body flow, I started using Gaiam's Body Pure Foot detox. I actually had some of these left over from when I used them months ago, so like the sauna this was an easy no-extra cost prep for me. My husband and I have used Gaiam's foot detox pads a couple of different times and felt they did a good job of helping the body cleanse itself, and left us feeling better. I started these on the Saturday before surgery and will continue them for two more days – I want to have whatever the foot pads bring out into my blood stream to be flushed out before surgery. Detox – Check, in progress.

As a last night-before prep, though really I should have started with this early, we have scheduled a massage for me to have the muscles loose, blood flowing, and my body ready for the next trauma (surgery). I should have started having one of these a week for the past month or so, however, time (oh and that money thing), I had not done this. We will either schedule one with a professional masseuse (or enlist my husband if that becomes necessary) the night before as a last minute fill-in if I need to, however my husband and I both believe in the power of regular massages for optimal health. (We're not in a position as of yet to schedule those, but I think it is a good thing and I have had massages when I could for body recovery and prep, especially before giving birth to my sons.) So massage – almost checked.

So, I was / am feeling a little more engaged in my own recovery – with little to thanks to the medical community. Would any of this help? And if it would, shouldn't I have been told all of this? Isn't surgery after all supposed to be about the patient outcomes, and doesn't the patient have a large role in that? Possibly some of that Western/Eastern medicine difference coming out?

Just to reiterate the disclaimer ...I have no medical training, and no scientific evidence or case studies to demonstrate a relationship between the pre-op prep steps I took and their impact on rhinoplasty outcome. I don't know that it would or did help, however it is my belief that the healthier and stronger the body is the better able it will be to deal with surgery and heal itself. Again, this is my personal surgery experience, not that of the medical community.

Thank you to the blogging community, my supportive husband, Rachel, Uncle Don and Aunt Karen, Dr. Fortier, and Dr. Caserma, my pre-op prep now consisted of:

- Bromelain
- Arnica (on reserve for post-op)
- Swiss Therapy Eye Mask (on reserve for post-op)
- In-Shape - Gaiam Cardio Wake-Up, Trainer Intervals, Shakeology
- Human Growth Hormone
- Sauna
- High Water Intake
- Chiropractic Care
- Gaiam Body Pure foot de-tox
- Massage

So, I have to be more ready... right? To my doctor's short list of three or four items I have added ten positive steps. I am taking control, practicing optimal health and empowering my recovery... right? This still feels inadequate. Why couldn't someone have given me a more holistic checklist of surgery preparation? And where does my mental/emotional state fit into all of this, because at this time I am nervous, anxious and antsy, which then messes with my muscle tension and my spine alignment. I Breathe... I tune into iTunes and play Ryan Starr's Breathe. (Or if that fails blow it all off with some good Jason Aldean, Tim McGraw, Van Halen or AC/DC.) Note to self – add, "Re-shuffle my iPod" to my pre-op To Do list.

So, with an additional ten items of prep started, completed, on-going or coming up, I should feel more empowered and stronger – like I have better odds of improving my surgery outcome.

One of the greatest barriers or challenges with surgery, as I see it, and with that whole disclaimer about slight chance of death, etc. put aside, is that when you enter the hospital, almost no matter what hospital that is and what level of care, once you submit to being in surgery or even just a patient, your status as an independent emotional / mental individual is ignored.

Following my knee surgery I couldn't order a simple piece of bread (not toast, not buttered, just bread) from the cafeteria even though I knew for me it was what my stomach would tolerate best and would be best for my body – the cafeteria couldn't figure out bread, only buttered toast.

After my hysterectomy, my doctor was able to get me a unit on the maternity wing – imitation hard wood floors, quiet private room, happy RNs, but I couldn't be released until my doctor cleared it – and my doctor didn't want to come in to clear me because she didn't have a babysitter so I sat in the hospital for hours waiting for my doctor's childcare to pull through, and wasn't that fun when all I wanted to do was go home and rest - which was supposedly the thing I needed most at the time.

While these hospital experiences could hardly rate as bad, the minute you walk into the hospital, your clothes, personal belongings and jewelry are taken away and you are issued a well-laundered pastel color open-backed hospital gown. The dreaded hospital gown. Millionaire or homeless, the hospital gown is the same. ICU coma patient or rhinoplasty outpatient, the hospital gown is the same - utterly demoralizing, no offense to the designers of such. And really, the problem is less with the gown itself than what it comes to represent from the patient's perspective – you, as the patient, have lost any control over yourself, you are in the hands of the doctor and the medical community now and are no longer a vested partner. Therein lies the problem with the hospital gown (that and the open back) – it is the loss of your own individuality, control and empowerment, that even an illusion of which would help motivate patients, in my non-medical opinion, to see themselves as a strong, empowered partner. Could a hospital give you a choice of colors so the patient feels they have some level of choice and control over their own outcome and destiny? Could there be different logistical designs based on your surgery needs? Really, couldn't I keep my underwear on?

I don't know, but in my own effort to further become a patient/partner (not patient partner) in a hospital system that does not want me to be one – to empower and optimize my own outcomes, after all they are _my_ outcomes, I am still looking for what else I can do. I feel like my physical prep is pretty much as good as I can get it without going back in time, I am, with four days left to go, focusing on my emotional and mental prep, though admittedly I don't know what exactly this means or should mean. Again, no darn checklist.

Being who I am, whether because I am female or it's just me, this means I ask, are my toes done? I had a pedicure about a month ago and have extended the pedicure by touching it up, but I can't touch up the cute flowers on my big toe. Plus, my current color is a bright, happy blue, though I can't help but feel I would heal better with a fresher, bright, happy pink. (I can't tell you how many hours I have debated this and how embarrassed I would be if I knew how long I have spent debating this. However, when the anesthesiology puts me under, I will be naked except for my toe paint.) I had planned on going and getting a new pedicure, but our budget got tighter last week than we had planned – both my husband and I are independently employed, so I am trying to save money and have rationalized with myself that really, my toe color will not effect my surgery outcome, but will it?

It also means, that on the off-chance that the medical community allows me to keep my underwear on – I mean it's a nose surgery – the knives should be at least two feet from my pubic area, what underwear am I going to wear, which means what bra am I going to wear. The other connected question is what clothes do I wear into the hospital, before they take them away and issue me my standard hospital gown? What you wear should be easy to get off and on, no jostling the surgery site, no hard coordination as I will probably still be slightly groggy, and no heals or wedges along that same line of thinking. While I do realize, in my rational moments, that these are all trivial questions overall, they have become none-the-less important to me as I try to exercise some level of control in a situation where I've been indirectly told I'm not supposed to have any control. But hello – my body, my life!

I did get my hair trimmed a week ago. Just to make sure I felt "good". A People Stylewatch magazine article references statistics that dressing better improves mood. Googling this, there are many articles and even organizations that confirm that looking better (and dressing better is certainly a part of that) improves mood, confidence and a feeling of being in control of your situation in general. I think the same holds true for surgery, though People didn't address this. I also had my eyelashes tinted and my bikini area waxed – not for the surgeon, for myself. I wasn't worried that anyone would look at me as anything other than a patient, however I wanted to feel as good as possible about myself going into this adventure.

So, back then to my debate over clothes and the color of my toes. These are items that remain unchecked. I'm assuming a button-up would be preferable to a shirt that I pull over my head as I don't want to bump my new nose, but I have received no guidance in this area, and frankly don't own any button-up shirts unless you're talking a business suit; I'm more of a jeans and tank top and cute little jacket kind of a girl, but I certainly don't want to wiggle into one of my tank tops with a swollen, sore face. Hmmm.... The debate continues.

I did start packing my "To-Go" bag for the hospital. We live 90 minutes from the hospital and the total surgery includes two pre-op appointments the afternoon before surgery, the surgery, and then one post-op the morning after. With four appoints in two days, two younger boys and a 90 minute drive, we decided to stay the night before my surgery and the night after at a hotel just over a mile from the hospital. My mom is flying in to watch the boys while I have my appointments and surgery and we made sure the hotel had a pool, walking access to a waterfront park and other easily accessible activities. As we are staying two nights away from home, and I have not been told what I need or what to anticipate, I started packing my To Go bag (as well as movies and swim suits, etc. for the boys).

As of now, 9:00pm four days before the surgery, my To Go bag includes Bromelain, arnica gel, arnica tablets, the eye masks, extra Carmex lip balm (those cold operating rooms are drying right, I can't have it on during surgery, but after?), dry shampoo and face cleaning wipes – in case I don't feel up to a whole shower but want to feel like a real person the next day, chicken noodle soup, saltine crackers, rice cakes, Gatorade, and sparkling mineral water – food alternatives since I don't know how I'll be feeling afterwards but want to be prepared and don't know where the nearest store will be or what is on the hotel's room service menu, as well as the liquids to keep myself hydrated. I also packed Bonine, a motion sick pill. I tend to get dizzy or lose my equilibrium more often than the average person. After my hysterectomy, the general anesthetics made me really dizzy, the Bonine seemed to make a noticeable difference very quickly. My husband also talked about bringing our humidifier since the hotels' usually have forced air that dries you out. Oh, and chocolate, I have a 74% Dagoba New Moon Dark Chocolate bar in my bag. Chocolate tends to help everything. Wonder if I should bring a bar for the doctors operating on me? Yep – that's the extent of my packing so far, based on my maniacal approach to optimizing my experience.

I made a list of the things I need to bring for my family and that will be easier to pack. But for me,

I feel like I'm stuck in a very feminine (and useless – or is it?) decision making disorder of what to pack – what clothes (slip on shoes not wedges or heals), shirt, underwear, bra, purse and toe nail polish. I had actually ordered a new bra and underwear for this occasion, but after receiving them the other day the sizing was slightly off. I'm trying not to take it as a bad sign that the bra was the wrong size, I probably won't have my toes painted and I can't find the purse I wanted to bring – three strikes is good right?

The surgery will surely go ahead whether I answer these questions or not, after all, they will issue me dreaded hospital gown regardless. However, I would like these questions answered. Not only that, I would like to feel good about the answers. I would like to feel prepared, strong, empowered – like I am helping my own healing even though I'm mostly unconscious on the operating table, or because I'm mostly unconscious on the operating table. Regardless of which it is, I wish the medical community (and medical bloggers) had readily available information to address the whole me so we can work together to achieve optimal outcomes. After all, they publish papers on their surgery stats, right? If my toe nail polish color might help improve their stats, should it be considered, its part of the patient preparation...?

What Is In My "To Go" Bag?

As I mentioned, since we live 90-120 minutes from OHSU where the surgery is being conducted, and I have a pre-op appointment the afternoon before and post-op appointment the morning after, we decided to stay in Portland two nights, arriving the day of my pre-op appointment. I made reservations at the Avalon Hotel and Spa (later renamed River's Edge Hotel and Spa) less than a mile from the hospital but along the Willamette River for some peace. (The Riverview Room was beautiful and perfectly met our needs, as did the amenities – fridge, microwave and separate master bedroom - and location of the hospital, though close, healthy, basic food turned out to be a bit of a challenge.)

My "to go" bag was then the essentials I need (or think I need or want to have just in case) for two nights. What I packed fell into three general categories: personal items (clothes, toiletries, etc.), post-op items (nasal spray, etc.) and general recovery items (food, etc.). I have to confess, while I pack extremely efficiently and light for business trips and vacations, I tend to pack more the less I know what to expect; as I felt I didn't know what to expect I may have over-packed somewhat.

My "to go" bag, technically one suitcase and a toiletry bag, included:

I. Personal Items.
   a. Pre-Op Work-Out Gear (I went running the night before my surgery)

       i. Shorts, Tank, Socks, Nikes

b. Nightgown (New Victoria's Secret gray-striped Mayfair flannel pajama set)

> *In Actuality...Loved these! Felt like my first "adult" pjs, practical but feminine too! Disclaimer is loved them so much I didn't want to get blood on them so I didn't wear them until a it was nearly a week post-op!*

c. My Surgery Outfit

       i. Easy on/off Sandals (no heels)

       ii. Underwear/Bra (both new from Victoria's Secret)

       iii.   An Easy Slip-on Dress (sundress from Cabi)

       iv.   Scarf (bright pink!)

       v. Carried my fedora for post-surgery

d. Day Two Outfit

       i. Slip on short wedges

       ii. Underwear/Bra

       iii.   Skirt

       iv.   Easy slip on Tank Top

       v. Scarf

> *In Actuality...I didn't wear the Day Two Outfit I packed. The tank felt like it was going to be challenge with my swollen, bandaged nose, and I was still a little wobbly so I thought better of the wedges. Instead I opted to re-wear my day of surgery outfit that I had only worn for an hour the day*

before.

e. Toiletries

    i. Neutrogena Deep Clean Oil-Free Makeup remover Cleansing Wipes

    ii. Face Soap for Night before

    iii. Shampoo/Cream Rinse for Night before – washed hair at last possible moment night before

    iv. Dry Shampoo

    v. Hair Dryer

    vi. Round brush

    vii. Water spray

    viii. Burt's Bees Milk & Honey Body Lotion – hospitals are dry, I put lots of lotion on my whole body before surgery and my hands and feet after surgery.

In Actuality...I went on total faith that I would not feel like I would not be able to be do make-up the morning after surgery and left my make-up bag at home! (I was told for morning of surgery you couldn't wear any make-up and I had made sure to get into the aesthetician and have my lashes tinted the week before surgery to help with the lack of mascara.) I'm one of those people who don't leave home without basic make-up so this was major – but I wouldn't have used it if I brought it.

f. Burt's Bees Beeswax Lip Balm and Carmex Moisturizing Lip Balm – I anticipated the dehydration from surgery would carry over and I used these both pre and post op.

g. My Stuffed Hedgehog – even grownups need a stuffed friend sometimes 💻①

h. iPod and Headset – I had downloaded some new music and re-organized my playlists.

    In Actuality...I didn't know exactly when I would use this, and ended up using it only during my run the night before, but I did bring it to the hospital in case... didn't use, but had it.

i. Kindle – I love to read and anticipated having some good reading time available during my recovery time. I downloaded a couple of books in anticipation of this reading time.

    In Actuality...I didn't use my Kindle, except for the night before as I was going to bed, but I had it and did use it at home the days following my surgery.

j. The Regular Stuff – purse, phone, phone charger, wallet with cash for hotel valet and for my husband to buy breakfast in the hospital cafeteria.

II.   Medical Items – I brought both the things I expected to need immediately after surgery, as well as those we had gathered for the week after to check in with the doctor, so these were not all items I needed immediately afterwards.

a. Prescription Antibiotics – to start the day after surgery

b. Prescription Pain Medications – to start the evening after surgery

In Actuality... I had asked the doctor what was the norm for taking the pain medication. He told me most people take them for the first three days, and then didn't need them anymore and there was actually very little pain associated with this surgery. He was right and I took the pain meds for the first three days after surgery but only twice a day – at nap time and night time consistent with my sleep patterns and I took them more for comfort while sleeping more than for the need to mask pain.

c. Swiss Therapy Eye Mask

d. Human Growth Hormone (with Needles and Car Cooler)

e. Extra Strength Tylenol – This was the post-prescription pain medication Dr. Power had advised me to get, I brought this just to "check our post-op prep" with the medical staff. *I did end up taking this off and on the three weeks following my surgery (after day three post-op – after I stopped taking the prescription pain medication.*

f. Arnica, Hylands 30 mg and Boiron Arnicare Arnica Cream - I brought these to "check our post-op prep" with the medical staff, as well as to use immediately following surgery.

In Actuality... I found out in my pre-op with Dr. Kim's assistant, Jeff, that I should (could) have been taking the arnica tabs starting 10-days pre-op. I wish I would have known that, but didn't, so I actually started taking the tabs in their office during my pre-op prep the afternoon before my surgery and continued with the tablets until two weeks after the surgery and have continued use of the Arnicare cream up until at least one month post-op (still using it at the time of this writing.)

g. Neilmed NasoGEL – Saline Spray. This was one of the items Dr. Power, in our pre-pre op call instructed me to have on reserve for after surgery.

In Actuality... I bought this brand because it was the same brand as the Nasal Wash that Dr. Smith gave me during our initial consultation for post-op. I bought two bottles of this. Dr. Kim's assistant gave me three bottles of Major Deep Sea Premium Saline. The biggest difference between the brands that I can tell is that NeilMed contains aloe and has a slimmer applicator point (much appreciated) and the Major Deep Sea Saline does not have aloe and has a much wider applicator point. I preferred the NeilMed and have – 30 days post-op used one bottle of the Major Deep Sea brand and six bottles of the NeilMed Nasal Spray. (My surgery was done during the dry summer months, which if you are scheduling your surgery is something you might want to consider, I think fall or spring, seasons with a higher humidity point, may be easier on the patient recovery – something else I didn't know pre-op to consider though I don't think it harmed my outcome, just less comfortable and I used more saline spray.) I also tried Arm & Hammer Simply Saline, but found the tip too big and the spray way too forceful for my sensitive post-op nose.

h. Neilmed Nasal Wash Kit– Dr. Smith gave me this during our initial consultation. I brought these to "check our post-op prep" with the medical staff, though I was told I would not need it for a couple of weeks post-op.

In Actuality... The result of coordinating two doctor involved in one surgery (or not coordinating them) (though I thought, leaders of their field working in the same office they would be in agreement). Dr. Smith gave it to me for post-op usage, Dr. Kim said I didn't need it. To date, one month post-op, I haven't used it, thought that's not to say I may some day....

i. Bromelain – I started taking this before my surgery as I mentioned in the pre-op and will continue to take this for a couple of weeks post-op.

j. Bonine – For my dizziness and to possibly use in the recovery room.

k. Pharmanex Nanopak Multi-Vitamins – As part of my normal health regimen and to maintain my general and pre-surgical well being.

III. General Recovery Items – this was mostly food and drinks. I didn't know what I would feel like but was anticipating that I would not feel very brave (sticking with bland, known foods rather than gambling on unknowns) with the anesthetics still in my system. *(And I was right, though my choices in the moment were a little different than I anticipated.)* I was also staying in a hotel for two days instead of being at home, so I tried to anticipate everything I would need being away from home.

a. Trader Joe's Mixed Berry Sparkling Water (Case!) – I was very focused on being hydrated before surgery and keeping hydrated afterwards, as this is something the research and blogs I found said were important and later confirmed by my doctor. So I drank a lot the night before and wanted to have it available for the next day as well. I brought 10 bottles (one was drunk on the car trip), I think I drank 5 in the two days I was there. (I didn't want to pack my Soda Stream, so the sparkling water was an easy alternative.)

b. Gatorade Powder – Along the same thinking of the sparkling water, I brought the Gatorade Powder to try to re-stabilize my body after the surgery as surgery itself can be harsh and I anticipated reacting to the anesthetics as well as being slightly being slightly dehydrated afterwards. This is also what I typically have when I have been nauseated in the past and my stomach is iffy, it can still hold it down. *(I drank two glasses of Gatorade the evening after my surgery.)*

c. Premium Saltine Crackers – These are of admittedly little nutritional value, but seem to help me with upset stomach, which I was anticipating. *I did end up eating a handful of these the evening after my surgery and the next morning.*

d. Progresso Chicken Noodle Soup. Going with the old adage that chicken noodle soup heals what ails you, this seemed like good recovery food. It also has a relatively high sodium content which is something my body tends to crave when I'm sick. *In Actuality... I didn't end up eating any, but I had packed it.*

e. Top Ramen Noodles – this was both for myself as well as the boys. Again, admittedly little to no nutritional value, but seem to be simple to digest and have relatively high sodium content that is helpful. *In Actuality... I didn't end up eating any, but I had packed it.*

f. Dagoba New Bar (74% Cacao) – a girl needs her chocolate right? And isn't high quality chocolate high in antioxidants? I don't know if it is or not, but this seemed like a wise item to pack. *In Actuality... I didn't end up eating any, but I had packed it, and had even offered a bar to my doctor before surgery, in case it would help his mood too.*

g. Chex-mix – another of my "go-to" foods when I'm sick or anticipating being sick; for some reason when I have a migraine coming on, salt seems to help kick it, and Chex-mix has to have one of the highest sodium counts, and is easy to transport. I take Chex-mix on flights with me. *In Actuality... I didn't end up eating any, but I had packed it.*

h. 32 ounce Starbucks Cup with Straw – When I was resting after the birth of each of my boys, having a glass with a straw was vital; I drank a lot more water when I wasn't as worried pouring it all over myself. *In Actuality... I ended up drinking the water out of the bottles rather than my cup with the straw, as I found it difficult to suck on the straw after my surgery, it hurt my nose.*

In Actuality... While I had carefully thought out the food I brought and thought I might want after my surgery, what I really wanted at the time – both before and after my surgery – turned out to be different than I anticipated. After my run the night before my surgery I had a massage. Between the run and my massage I had no desire to have anything with preservatives or processed foods. While my family had Spaghetti Factory that night I had salad and fruit. The evening and mornings after my surgery followed suit and I mostly had fruit, though I also ended up having some saltines both meals after surgery (dinner the night of surgery and breakfast the morning after).

Pre-Op Prep: Eight Hours and Counting

Prepping for my nose surgery, I was nervous, felt totally unprepared to embark such an... adventure... journey... undertaking. Ok, the doctors told me they would take care of everything, so really, I'm just expected to follow a basic list of things not to do, show up, change into a hospital gown and let them stick me with an IV. After that, the medical profession seems to hold that I sleep through the rest and the medical professionals – the doctors and surgical team will make me breathe again. However, it's not that simple to me, nor am I okay with that version of what were the coming events.

So, I had spent 30 days prepping for my surgery. My prep list was created from personal experience, personal beliefs, and some research. This was my prep though "and may not represent the opinions of the medical community." Sorry, felt I had to add that. I'm not sure if what I did changed my outcomes at all or if there was more or different that I really should have done, though I have to believe it has benefitted me.

My prep consisted, in short, of:
- Bromelain
- Arnica (on reserve for post-op)
- Swiss Therapy Eye Mask (on reserve for post-op)
- In-Shape - Gaiam Cardio Wake-Up, Trainer Intervals, Shakeology
- Human Growth Hormone
- Sauna
- High Water Intake
- Chiropractic Care
- Gaiam Body Pure foot de-tox
- Massage

I thought this felt somewhat holistic and though possibly overkill, it was all I could think of and I still felt unprepared. The hospital had scheduled my pre-op appointments - one with the doctor and one with the hospital surgical staff – for the afternoon before my appointment. The appointments could have been made at another time however they were accommodating my travel schedule and did not feel an earlier appointment would be any more beneficial. So the night before I'm going to be told how to prep and what to expect.

I was heading up to Portland from Corvallis (a two hour drive) the morning before my surgery. We found a hotel that could accommodate my family's needs and would spend the night before and night of the surgery at the hotel, so we could also see the doctor the morning after for my first post-op check-up.

However, I was not really comfortable. I still didn't feel like I knew what I needed to do – not just for myself at this point, but also taking into account my children and their needs and my husbands. My mom had agreed to come help watch the kids and we were meeting her in Portland the day before my surgery. But what of after – entertainment for the kids, food for the family? I wanted to try to ensure I had all of my errands run and the kids planned for so my husband and family felt the least impacted. I knew I would need prescriptions, but what and who was going to go get those? When? I felt I needed to talk to the doctor to prep for my prep.

So three days before my surgery, some telephone tag ensued and I was able to connect with a very patient Dr. Powers, Dr. Smith's Physician Assistant. She patient answered my questions in what did I need to do to prep for after the surgery – according to them. She:

- Ordered two prescriptions: Antibiotics, pain medication
- Included in my supplies to get:
  - Afrin
  - Extra Strength Tylenol
  - Saline Nose Spray (no brand requested)
  - Nasal Wash Kit (which the doctor had given us when we first met with him)

I tried to push the conversation to see what else I needed to do to prep the rest of me, besides my nose, but was assured they would take care of the rest. And, I do believe them – as far as the surgery was concerned. We sought out and partnered with a highly competent team of doctors. I had not worries about the surgery itself, or at least their roles in my surgery – this was not nervousness about their skills, though I have to confess I'm always nervous about the skills of the anesthesiologist! This was more about the total outcome of the surgery. (I could just be a control freak. I have been told I'm rather demanding as a boss.)

Anyway, as a good patient I ran out and picked up prescriptions and the other supplies. I also did end up getting that pedicure – I went with bright pink (with flowers on the big toes) to match my new bright pink, grey and orange purse and matching bright pink scarf (with a new bra and undies underneath). This completed what I had decided on as my "day of surgery outfit". Ok, not a big milestone in surgery prep for the medical community, but I did feel better. I was packed, my toes were pretty, I had gotten the last minute pre-pre prep words of wisdom from the doctors, packed the car and was um ...ready to go...?. As a last minute thought, my husband grabbed my rain fedora on the way out the door. (Only noting because it came in handy!)

At 3:30 p.m. on August 8th, after settling into the hotel and squaring the kids away with grandma, my husband and I checked-in for our pre-op appointment with Dr. Kim. (While our initial consultation was scheduled with Dr. Smith, the surgery required work by both Dr. Smith and Dr. Kim, but as Dr. Kim's work was more extensive, Dr. Kim took the lead in my pre and post-op appointments.) Dr. Kim's assistant (sorry Jeff, I don't know your actual title!) led us into the patient room, reviewed my chart, sprayed industrial Afrin up my nose and walked us through some of the prep and post for the next day. My husband and I had also come prepared with our prep list and the supplies Dr. Power instructed us to get. Jeff added to our list of post-surgery needs. He told us we would need another Swiss Therapy Mask, though what we bought had been perfect, two bags of frozen peas, and nail polish remover. He also said _not_ to use the Afrin post-surgery as Dr. Power had instructed and that we would also not need the nasal wash kit that Dr. Smith had given us. Dr. Kim's assistant also provided us with another bottle of nasal saline spray. We reviewed our prep list with Jeff, who confirmed we did everything right, expect... I should have been taking the Arnica for at least 10 days before my surgery instead of just having on hand for after. I didn't think your body would store the arnica, however it does, so that is something it would have been nice to know, that I would have done, but didn't since I didn't know! Finding that out was a little disheartening, as it was something I had on hand and could have easily done, but didn't. I started downing arnica tabs right that minute as we were talking! We also asked if, since moisture was such a big thing in helping heal after nose surgery, should we have a humidifier. (My husband had dried ours out to bring with us to the hotel, but we left on the bathroom floor at our house, after all, who brings a humidifier to a hotel for a two-night stay?) We were told the humidifier would not be good.

That was the end of pre-pre-op prep two. On to our actual pre-op prep appointment with Dr. Kim. Dr. Kim is always reassuring and confident, his assessments thorough but not time consuming. Dr. Kim came in with three med students who all witnessed my pre-op appointment. (I found that I didn't mind having med students at all of my appointments with me, though it is a curious feeling to be "watched" as a patient. I found myself checking my reactions.)

Dr. Kim examined my nose and asked what questions we had. My husband and I felt we understood the actual surgery and had little questions about that aspect. (My husband and I are fairly comfortable in general with trusting experts to be experts in areas beyond our areas of experience or knowledge, and rhinoplasty is out our areas of expertise and we believe in the surgeons we chose.) As with our discussion with Jeff, we asked about pre-op preparation. The only area that differed from what Jeff instructed us on was the humidifier, Dr. Kim felt this would be very beneficial. Beyond that, Dr. Kim was ready for surgery and felt we were as well. (I think he was a little amused by our level of prep and desire to be "prepared" as surgery is his domain, not ours, but he humored us as an indulgent parent would.)

My final pre-op appointment of the day was with the hospital's surgery unit. Here they reviewed my basic medical history, took blood samples, checked my blood pressure, pulse, listened to my lungs and made a few notes for the next day. One of the more important outcomes of this meeting, at least to me, was the review of my prior surgery recovery. We discussed my dizziness, asked out having Bonine available for post-surgery recovery. The med tech said to talk to the recovery unit in the morning, but that Bonine should be fine. She also made a note to give me a scopolamine patch before surgery. This appointment was pleasant enough, lasting only about 20 minutes. There were no additional pre-op instructions, save the do not eat after midnight instruction.

After leaving the pre-op appointments, I was nervous and anxious, not ready for tomorrow, battling to not feel dread, and just trying to relax. Did I mention the whole surgery thing makes me really uncomfortable and general anesthesiology really nervous? I'm sure that came up earlier. You hear those horror stories about people dying under general anesthesiology or about people who were never quite "under" and were tortured at being awake and feeling the agony and pain but unable to relay their living nightmare to the surgical team. To be fair, I know these are really, really, really rare instances overly sensationalized by the media; that in actuality thousands of surgeries are performed across the country every day and are complete "non-events." However, this is one of my personal fears.

So, after leaving the hospital, I hurriedly changed into my running gear, grabbed my iPod and went for a 2-mile run along the waterfront. The scenery was beautiful, my newly restocked iPod a comfort, and the run was a proactive, mental reaffirmation that I was taking positive steps and somewhat (maybe) in control of my own well being. Between my last pre-op appointment and the massage I had scheduled, I didn't have a lot of time, so my run was actually a little shorter than I would have liked, but felt really good and I am glad I did it.

After my run, a quick shower and then down to my massage. (Meanwhile, my husband and kids were running around Portland trying to find the nearest store or pharmacy to gather the missing post-op recovery items mentioned by Dr. Kim and his staff during our pre-op appointment.) Ninety-minutes of quiet relaxation and massage – aaahhhh. There were a number of massage types available from deep tissue work to detox massages. I asked for a general reflexology, but nothing too deep. Whatever toxins were in my muscles at this point, with only hours until surgery, I didn't want my body to be in recovery before I even got into surgery. I have to say, the massage felt really good; though I don't think I've ever had a massage that didn't feel good.

A healthy dinner, a long shower to relax and wash my hair, some good "down-time" with my husband and boys followed by more Arnica. Supposedly I'm ready. Wow, I so don't feel it. And wow, I don't think sleep is coming anytime soon. Off to bed, tomorrow is my surgery.

Recovery: On to the Hard Part

So, the dreaded green hospital gown, while still dreaded, was actually purple and came with an attached heater and heater hose and a pair of matching purple socks - still backless though. My hospital admission and surgery prep was uneventful and everyone we talked to - the many, many people we talked to - were very helpful, warm and sincere. Off to groggy-land and asleep I went. I had a horrific moment of panic as they wheeled me away from my husband, but luckily the drugs had started kicking in and it was short-lived.

Waking up after the surgery, the first thing I remember was the voices of nurses in recovery and the beeps of machinery. Before my eyes were even open, the next thing I felt was an overwhelming need to vomit, I sat up and told them I was going to be sick. Welcome back to the land of the conscious. Luckily I remember little of the next few hours. Eventually I was returned to my pre-op room for recovery and my husband was able to stay with me. I was inordinately dizzy, to the point that the hospital staff started getting concerned. They told me that after surgery, I could expect to leave the hospital within 2-3 hours; with surgery scheduled for 9:00am, we anticipated being back at the hotel between 1-3 depending on how long the surgery took. In actuality, with the amount of dizziness and vomiting I experienced, we did not return to the hotel until after 6:00pm. I mostly ended up leaving the hospital on pure will - I was not really feeling any better, but I was not going to be admitted for the night!

I received plenty of odd looks coming back to the hotel with gauze and tape over my nose and a modified mouth mask holding additional gauze to my nose. I'm sure I looked as awful as I felt. I made it up to our room, only needing to stop and rest twice along the way. Luckily the dizziness and vomiting subsided by later that night with the help of Bonine, Gatorade and saltine crackers. As expected, I did not feel like showering or being up and around that night. I took the time to reassure my boys and change into a sleeping shirt. After that, I had my first food of the day - fruit and saltines, began the 20-minute cycles of using the eye masks, took Bonine, a pain pill and went to sleep. Part of the immediate recovery key, I was told, was to start using the Swiss Therapy Eye masks almost immediately and to continually use them as much as possible during the first 24-72 hours post-surgery. A little hard to continually change them while you're sleeping, however my husband was really great about making sure this happened that first night and the days following, often getting little sleep himself so I could continue with the packs.

You are also supposed to sleep nearly upright the first week after surgery, but with your head tilted back. We were able to arrange the pillows to be mostly upright and mostly comfortably, but if I knew this in advance, I probably would have researched and bought one of those shaped sitting pillows or a beanbag or something to make this easier - the pillows tend to slip and mush down over time.

The morning after my surgery, I had my first post-op follow-up with Dr. Kim. He thought the surgery went well and I looked good. He changed the dressing and looked in my nose. Then, we were good to go. We checked out of the hotel and drove back to Corvallis. The 90-mile ride home was not my most comfortable ride, though it rated higher than driving to the birthing center in active labor. A tip - wearing sunglasses after surgery is not an option, your nose is much to sensitive (maybe those old-people wrap-around films would have worked) and the sun felt extra bright with the medication, so a baseball hat would have been helpful; I had my fedora which helped some, but the brim is not big enough to help shield the sun from your eyes. Also, one of those air travel pillows that you blow up for sleeping on airplanes and looks like a "C" might have been helpful for making my head comfortable.

The next couple of days passed with regularity. My nose, for the most part, didn't truly hurt, it was more uncomfortable and felt constantly on edge, like you had to sneeze but didn't actually sneeze. I did take pain medication through the first two days, but mostly for sleep, after that, Extra-Strength Tylenol took enough of the edge off to work. My nose continued to drain and bleed some for the next four days. We changed the gauze regularly and used the modified face mask the hospital gave us to hold the gauze in place - though after one day of use, the mask started really bothering my ears, it worked better than anything else we found so I kept using it.

By day two I started being able to move around the house, read my Kindle and function relatively normally, though much slower and I didn't bend over or put my nose below my torso. My first shower was a little bit of a challenge, but felt great and my husband dried my hair for me, since flipping my head over to blow dry it was not an option. I found that my nose was much more uncomfortable rather than actual painful. And while I could breath immediately better after surgery than before, my nose started getting more and more stuffed feeling in the days after the surgery. (I found out later that this was primarily dried blood caught in the shunts that had been placed in each of my nostrils. Once they removed these, one week after surgery, I was immediately able to breath better.) The big tape and gauze on my nose felt very clumsy and cumbersome, though it was really of little impact.

By day three I stopped taking the prescription pain medicate, though I started taking the Extra Strength Tylenol. Each day was a little easier than the previous one and each day there was less blood. I felt a little stronger and could do more each day.

My second post-op appointment was one week after surgery. At this appointment, Jeff removed the surgical tape from my nose (yeah!) and Dr. Kim removed the shunts. after spraying my nose with saline and examining the interior and exterior surgical points, Dr. Kim removed the shunts from my nose - one from each nostril. And wow was that an eye-shutting experience! First, the shunts are much larger than you would ever imagine would fit in your nose. Second, the process is vaguely reminiscent of a doctor removing a baby with forceps from the birthing canal. Okay, not nearly as painful, though I did squeeze my husband's hand pretty good during the removal, but the process is much the same. Dr. Kim reached the clamp way up my nose and gently-ish pulled the shunt out of nostril. The shunt was approximately two inches long and almost half an inch wide - apparently there is a lot of space in your upper nasal cavity; the only problem is you have to pass the shunt appropriate for the larger cavity through the smaller lower cavity. It was an uncomfortable process and mildly painful, though it was thankfully over quickly. My nose was oily, pores really dirty and still fairly swollen, but I could breathe and was assured my nose was recovering wonderfully and would continue to recover over the next year.

Four days later my family left on a three week driving vacation to California. My nose was still uncomfortable and swollen, though not noticeably to people who didn't know me, however I could breathe and was could function almost fully. I was still taking Tylenol, though only when needed now, no longer continually, and being very careful with my nose.

Traveling after Rhinoplasty: What I Know Now, What I Wish I Would Have Known

My recovery was fairly typical I think – I stopped the prescription pain medication three days after surgery, used Extra Strength Tylenol off and on. Nine days after having rhinoplasty surgery for a deviated septum, my family and I went on a road trip. While idea of taking a vacation immediately following minor surgery may not occur to everybody as the best idea, it was how it worked out for me. We (my husband, two boys – ages 7 and 9, and I) left Corvallis, Oregon on a road trip to Southern California to visit family and friends. We were coordinating our vacation schedule with the schedules of various friends and family members so our options for scheduling our vacation were fairly narrow. We knew going into my nose surgery that we had vacation scheduled soon after, and we could have moved my surgery, but then it was going to start pushing into my kids' school schedule and my work schedule, so between the complexity of scheduling our family vacation and our own time frames, we kept both activities as scheduled. What that meant to me however, I knew very little about. What would traveling while recovering from rhinoplasty be like? How would I feel 2 days after surgery? One week? One month?

During our pre-op appointment, Dr. Kim said that after the first week, the swelling and bruising around my nose and eyes should mostly be gone, and that by the end of the second week, most people would not be able to tell that I had surgery, that only those who knew me well would be able to tell that my nose was still swollen and that the surgical scars would not be very visible. I was also told that the nasal swelling could take up to one year to fully go down. My post-op instructions from Dr. Kim also said not to sneeze with your mouth close, vomit or expose yourself to high temperatures. The post-op instructions from the hospital surgical staff, told me not to lift anything heavier than a one-gallon milk container for up to two weeks and then begin to slowly reintroduce normal activities.

Ok – I can do that. But how would I feel and what would I feel like doing? I realize the medical staff cannot tell patients exactly how they will feel as everyone is different and every patient has a different life style and heals differently, but it would have been nice to know how some people did. I was able to find on Google images pictures of people post-rhinoplasty, but I don't know what the time frames were or how they felt. And then on top of that, if how did/would they have handled vacation one week post-op?

We left Corvallis on the afternoon of August 18th. Late summer in the Pacific Northwest and into California it was hot and dry! With temps in the low 90s and humidity 0 degrees, we were either driving with the air conditioning on (which is dehydrating) or at a rest stop in the dry heat. Either way, I used my nose spray and arnica cream nearly constantly, as well as my supply of Kleenex to then mop up my constantly dribbling nose. During the pre-op appointment with Dr. Kim, both Dr. Kim and his assistant Jeff highlighted the necessity of keeping your nose "well hydrated" – that moisture was one of the keys to recovery. I had slept with a humidifier in my bedroom every night since the surgery and had one going at the house full time, as I did on most of the vacation, but late-summer being outside or on a road trip; this was more of a challenge. If someone asked me, and they had the flexibility, I think I would advise considering scheduling rhinoplasty in spring or fall when the temperature is a little lower and humidity a little higher.

So, anyway, it's a hot, dry 17-hour, two-day drive from Corvallis to Southern California, and I used lots of saline spray and arnica cream! Also, keep the Extra Strength Tylenol handy. It's not something I needed constantly at this point, but when you need it, you need it. The lack of it being easily accessible literally drove my husband to exit the freeway, dig around in our luggage and find it, and then hold me as I was taking it as I cried at him out of frustration, dryness and general yuck. If I had been able to hold off the crisis with handy Tylenol, my husband (and kids) would have been spared a crying jag and my nose would have been spared an extra blowing.

In addition to being hot, dry 17-hour drive, it is also a bright two-day drive. Sunglasses are my norm; however they are not comfortable on a recovering rhinoplasty nose. At this time (30-days post surgery) they are still not comfortable on my nose for more than 5-10 minutes. At the time of our trip, I could only tolerate them for 1-3 minutes and then needed 20 or so minutes to recover before I could put them on again. Overall, this made sunglasses impractical for our drive. A baseball cap would have been great. And I meant to grab one... but in the final packing missed it. I did have my fedora, but the brim is just different. A baseball cap is a must post-surgery if you are a sunglass person and it is a sunny season. While I don't normally wear hats – I own two – this would have really helped!

My Outcomes

It has now been one year since my surgery, so what did we achieve and where am I today?

At six months, I would have said the surgery was 100% a success, today, I would decrease the success rate to 80%. Dr. Smith and Dr. Kim both advised me that one of the risks would be that more than surgery might be needed, or that the outcomes may change over time. While I'm not looking for a second surgery, I believe some of the blockage has regrown internally - I can no longer take a deep breathe in through my left nostril, there is an obstruction to the air flow. Having said that, it is much, much better than it was and we are not looking to redo the surgery... unless it regresses to where it was, then we would have to re-assess. But we'll jump off that bridge if we get to it.

With my breathing largely cleared, my body has rebalanced its natural circadian rhythm. I am also sleeping naturally, without prescription sleep aides and I am learning to "breathe" again. Amazingly, after not breathing naturally through my nose for nearly 20 years, this actually does take practice and after a year, I am still working on it, though it has gotten easier.

Physically, my nose is still sensitive to touch, but just at the tip. I have converted to wearing sunglasses with plastic lightweight frames with integrated nosepieces, as they do not put as much pressure on my nose. (I had to try a couple of pairs before I was able to get to one that worked - thank you Sunglass Hut for working with me and for your awesome return policy!)

I consider my surgery a success and better prepared for any medical interventions in the future, though I am certainly working hard to avoid those!

I still think as a training for doctors, each doctor should be made to strip, put on a hospital gown and attend a lecture on being patient focus while dressed in only the beloved hospital gown, may provide them with a different perspective! Maybe even have them stuck with an IV - the whole process - ick!

If you are considering rhinoplasty or any other surgery, I would encourage you to make sure you have complete confidence in your surgical team and have great staff around you. I think the team I had made a huge difference on my outcomes, though I do feel that if we would have worked together on pre-op procedures - even receiving a handout or booklet, it would have improved my experience and outcomes. I would also encourage you to put yourself in control of your own surgery. Yes, the surgeon and surgical team are the experts and will take care of the pieces and parts they are operating on, but that piece or part is only one small part of the total body and your experience, and the total body goes through the surgery, not just the incision site. Whatever the surgery, remember you are in charge of your body and your outcomes are as much your responsibility as your doctor's.

I hope this helps you on your journey!